I0457676

THE BOOK OF ETHICS
道德经

THE BOOK OF ETHICS

道 德 经

(TAO TE CHING)

The Original Art Of Living Inner Strength

Lao Tzu

老 子

Translated by

Tham Trong Ma

THE BOOK OF ETHICS

All rights reserved

First Edition

© Tham Trong Ma, 2022

CONTENTS

A Few Words

This book should not be considered a book of ideas or one giving the difference between the forces of good or evil or the distinction between right and wrong. However, while it may touch on these subjects, those are not the foundation upon which this book is written. This should be considered a book of timeless principles that have been practiced for thousands of years. A personal study has been done on the principles inherent in this book, and the result has been outstanding. But it should also be known that as much as this book is generally available for everyone who wants to read it, it is not meant for everyone. Some may find problems understanding the concepts explained within the pages or the nuggets of wisdom that may be hidden to a layman due to writing style. To enjoy this book and the treasure within, one must bare their minds and give a critical view to the words, for the words are not just made up. Every line has a purpose.

This book is divided into two parts: the *Way* and the *Virtue*. While these two elements may seem mutually exclusive, to some extent, they are also similar. And this book is here to offer insights into them.

Some scholars have considered *Tao Te Ching (The Book of Ethics)* to be a compilation of various sayings; even the text authorship, date of compilation, and date of composition have been greatly debated. These subjects are still being debated even today. Researchers are working tirelessly to gather the facts, but this mystery might continue for many generations to come. However, there is no doubt that the book – or a major part of it, as the case may be – is hugely credited to Lao Tzu. And until a different fact emerges about the true authorship of *The Book of Ethics*, Lao Tzu will continue to be known as the original author, which is most probably the truth anyway.

The oldest version of the book was dated as far back as the 4th century BC, when it was reported to have been excavated. However, some other dates emerged concerning the historical appearance of the book. Some have claimed that some parts of the text have been compiled later than the earliest portion of the *Zhuangzi*. A controversial manuscript about the *Tao Te Ching* inked on silk, which was reported to have been written in the 2nd century BC, has also been unearthed from Mawangdui.

The Book of Ethics is regarded as a fundamental text for philosophical and religious Taoism; indeed, it has strongly influenced other Chinese philosophy and religion schools. It also has a great influence on Legalism, Buddhism, and Confucianism. The text was largely translated and interpreted through the use of the Taoist concept when it was first introduced to China. Such professionals like artists, painters, poets, calligraphers, and gardeners have used *The Book of Ethics* as their source of inspiration.

Over the years, the book's influence has spread widely beyond the shores of East Asia; and it has held the title as one of the most translated works in world literature. It is no surprise that it has been translated into many widely spoke languages all over the world.

In the title, Tao Te Ching, *Tao* means 'way' in English or any of its close synonyms. However, the term was later extended to mean "the Way". This term, *Tao*, and its meaning were later adopted by other Chinese philosophers such as Hanfeizi, Mozi, Mencius, and Confucius. The word, and its meaning, has its concept in Taoism, where it implied the essential process of the universe.

However, the *Te* in *Tao Te Ching* means 'virtue' which, of course, has further meanings with 'inners strength,' 'personal character,' or 'integrity'. Modern terms have also chosen it to mean 'goodness' or 'moral excellence'.

Now from the two words, the term *tao-te* means 'ethical principles', 'morality', 'morals', or 'ethics'. Then *ching* also has its own meaning, which, in this context, is 'great book', 'classic', or 'canon'; hence the general title *The Book of Ethics* - or, if to be named more appropriately, should be titled *The Great Book of Ethics*, but we feel *The Book of Ethics* is appropriate; there should be no reason for verbosity since everyone who has read it has agreed that it is indeed a great book.

Tao Te Ching can also be given other synonymous titles, such as *The Classic of the Way's Virtues, The Book of the Way and of Virtue,* or *The Book of the Tao and Its Virtue.* Some translations have been titled *The Tao and its Characteristics; The Classic Book of Integrity and the Way; The Canon of Reason and Virtue;* and *A Treatise on the Principle and Its Action.*

As everyone familiar with it knows, *The Book of Ethics* has a long and complex textual history. It has been claimed to have dated back to two millennia, including silk, paper, and bamboo manuscripts discovered in the twentieth century.

The original *Tao Te Ching* is a short text that contains not more than five thousand Chinese characters in 81 brief chapters; the structure has been carefully followed in this translation. However, there is some evidence that the chapter divisions later had some additions simply for the sake of commentary or as an aid for easier memorization. Besides all the adulterations, revisions, translations, and abridgments, the original text was still more fluidly organized. There was the *Tao Ching* that begins from chapter 1 to chapter 37, and followed by *Te Ching,* which continues from chapters 38 to chapter 81.

As you will soon notice, even in this translation, the writing style is somehow concise and mysterious. All in all, the style is poetic. So while reading, you may feel that you are reading poetry. It is easy to get lost in the stanzas and lines, but the message will be fully received if you pay careful attention to the text. The writing style combines two major strategies –

the first strategy creates memorable phrases, and the second forces the reader to reconcile supposed contradictions in the general work.

The original version, written in Chinese characters, contained three writing styles: the first style is in the *zhuànshū* (seal script) form; then another version was written in *lìshū* (clerical script) and then finally *kǎishū* (regular script). These three styles have been maintained over millennia.

There have been many transmitted editions of *Tao Te Ching*, but there are three primary editions named after early commentaries. The first is the 'Yan Zun Version', which is just the extant of *Te Ching*, derives from a commentary attributed to Han dynasty scholars that went by the name Yan Zun. Then the second version is the 'Heshang Gong Version', which is named after the legendary Heshang Gong who lived during the reign of Emperor Wen of Han. The third version is the 'Wang Bi Version', which has a more verified origin than either the Yan Zun or the Heshang Gong. The man Wang Bi was a famous Three Kingdoms period philosopher on the *Tao Te Ching* and the *I Ching.*

In 1973, archeologists discovered copies of early Chinese books, known as Mawangdui Silk Texts, in a tomb dating from 168 BC. The texts have been associated with *Tao Te Ching*. Also, in 1993, the oldest known version of *Tao Te Ching*, written on bamboo tablets, was found in another tomb near the town of Guodian in Jingmen Hubei, and the text was dated before 300 BC. The Guodian Chu Slips has about 800 slips of bamboo with a total of 13,000 characters; 2,000 of those characters correspond with the *Tao Te Ching*.

The text in *The Book of Ethics* has thematic concerns with the Tao, otherwise known as 'Way', and how it is expressed by virtue. The book talks specifically about the virtues of naturalness and inaction, or non-action, as specifically referred to in the text.

Tao Te Ching has been translated over 250 times into Western languages, most of which are English, French, and German. According to Holmes Welch, "It is a famous puzzle which everyone would like to feel he had solved." It is hard to determine when *Tao Te Ching* was first translated to English, but the first English translation was publicly produced by John Chalmers, a Scottish Protestant missionary. He titled the book *The Speculation on Metaphysics, Polity, and Morality of the "Old Philosopher" Lau-size*.

However, translating *Tao Te Ching* didn't come easily to people; there were challenges. Since the text was written in ancient Chinese characters, some people had difficulty identifying some words' meanings. They only had to rely on the thematic approach of the general lines in the chapters before they could use suitable words to replace the ones they couldn't understand. Also, because there are no punctuation marks in Classical Chinese, it was difficult to determine where one sentence ended and where another began. So generally, it can be impossible to understand some chapters without moving sequences of characters from one place to another.

This particular translation has been made in the most straightforward and understandable way possible. I hope that you find this translation highly satisfying and refreshing.

About Lao Tzu

According to *History*, a book written by Tư Mã Thiên, Lao Tzu was from Khúc Nhân village, Khổ district, country of Sở. His family name was Lý, and his name is Nhĩ. He decided to rename himself Bá Dương and his nickname was Đàm. In his early days, he worked as a library keeper for the Zhou kingdom. It is predicted that he was born in 601 BC and resided in seclusion in 531 BC; he was 70 years old at that time.

According to legend, Lao Tzu was tired of the contemporary government, so he resigned from the library and rode the buffalo to hide. When he was passing through the gate, he met Doãn Hỷ, who was the gatekeeper at Hàm Cốc. Doãn Hỷ pulled him back and said: If you decide to stay in hiding, please write something for our descendants so that they may know what is happening in our world this time. Lao Tzu decided to put the gatekeeper's request into consideration. He stayed at the gate of Hàm Cốc and wrote the book called *The Book of Ethics* (Tao Te Ching). When he finished writing, he handed the book over to Doãn Hỷ and went into hiding. Since then, no one knows how and where he lived or died.

The only book Lao Tzu ever wrote was *The Book of Ethics*. This book was later divided into two parts consisting of 81 chapters. Part one has 37 chapters, talking about the Way and the second part has 44 chapters, talking about the Virtue. With a total of 5250 words in 1745 sentences, Lao Tzu denied and deconstructed the whole scale and organized the face of contemporary feudal society to construct a "non-existent" doctrine. *The Book of Ethics* advises people to live in harmony with nature, harmony with the universe, transform themselves and give up desire. He explained that if people and nature were in harmony, they would all be inanimate and desireless, so there was no need to fight and conquer. Therefore, humans will have peace, well-being, and happiness.

According to scholars today, *The Book of Ethics* is a spiritual book for those who follow the mystical and transcendent path. But objectively, one must recognize that the book is, first of all, a book written to urge the rulers and politicians to use the Way to rule the country. Lao Tzu was a sage who tried to bring ethics into politics, using his spiritual experiences to form a philosophical system.

Lao Tzu in *The Book of Ethics* also did not forget to advise politicians that if they know the Way, they do not need to take humanity, righteousness, courtesy, and wit to teach the people, just making them keep their simplicity with nature. The ideal society for Lao Tzu was a small country with few people. There was no need for deception, no need for civilization, no need for soldiers, no need for traffic, no need for luxury items. As long as one can eat fully, dress warmly, live peacefully, keep the custom of being gentle and courteous. So in chapter 80, he advised:

Food is simple but delicious.

Cloth is rudimentary but beautiful

The house is primitive but peaceful

Tradition is pure but fun

Lao Tzu is considered a semi-legendary figure in the entire Asian community. He was often portrayed as the contemporary of the powerful Confucius. However, some modern historians believed that Lao Tzu lived during the Warring States period of the 4th century BC; one could argue that it was the politics of war that inspired him to write the single book he wrote. The book, however, has been considered one filled with a lot of symbolism and deep meaning. Even Lao himself mentioned in his book that many people do not understand him and do not understand his teaching, so they do not know him. Even in his lifetime, before he left to live a life of isolation, Lao was often considered a strange person because of how he talked. He rarely spoke directly; most of his words were laced with deep meanings that required even deeper thoughts to understand, which is reflected in his writing. He was regarded as a sage (a very wise man).

It is hard to mention central figures of the Chinese culture and not mention Laozi. He was claimed by both the emperors of the Tang dynasty and the modern people who have the Li as their original surname; these *Li* people often considered Lao Tzu as the founder of their lineage. The accuracy of this claim, however, is only speculative.

Even after thousands of years since it was written, Laozi's work is still being embraced by Chinese legalism and various anti-authoritarian movements.

A consensus emerged around the mid-twentieth century when some scholars claimed that Lao Tzu's history is doubtful and that *Tao Te Ching* does not refer to a single individual. Some claimed it to be a Taoist compilation of sayings written by many hands. The oldest text of the *Tao Te Ching* that has so far been recovered as part of the Guodian Chu Slips. The text was written on the slips of bamboo around the late 4th century BC.

The *Tao Te Ching*, according to some other scholars, was an otherwise name for Laozi. It has been considered the source and ideal of all existence. The theme of the writing is to lead students to return to their natural state in harmony with Tao.

A lot of people have been influenced by Laozi and his work. They have advocated a restrained approach to statecraft and humility in leadership, either for tactical ends or for ethical and pacifist reasons. On another hand, however, various anti-authoritarian movements have accepted the teachings of Laozi on its emphasis on the power of the weak.

In an article for the *Encyclopædia Britannica* of 1910, Peter Kropotkin considered Laozi as among the earliest proponents of anarchist concepts. In the same vein, David Boaz of the Cato Institute took a passage from *Ta-Te Ching* and included it into his 1997 book titled *The Libertarian Reader*. But a philosopher such as Roderick Long believed that libertarian themes in Taoist perspectives are originally from earlier Confucian writers.

PART I

The Way

道

1

The Way[1] that can be spoken of is not the way of truth
A name[2] that can be called is not an eternal one

Anonymity is before heaven and earth Having a name is the mother of all species

When we are nonbeings, we infer mystery
And when we are beings, we recognize the quintessence[3]
The two elements mentioned above have the same origin But contain different names

They both have depth
The kind that is deep in the deepest level
That is the door to the occult.

2

Under the dome:
We know the beautiful because there is the ugly
And we know the good because there is the evil

Being and non-being that are born together
Are sometimes difficult and easy to complement
each other
Long and short are often compared together
High and low lean together
Sound and voice mingle together
Before and after also chase each other[4]

So according to the sages:
Act without moving
Teach without using words
Everything is spontaneous and can self-destruct

Create, but do not take over
Do, but do not count on
Succeed, then withdraw
Therefore, do not lose.

3

Do not respect the meek,
Make people not fight.
Do not make the rare precious,
Make people not steal.
Do not provoke desire,
Make people not confused.[5]

Rules of the saint:
Make people's mind empty, but fill their stomachs
Weaken the heart and soul, but make the bone
strong
This often makes people mindless without desire
So intellectualists do not dare to bother
There is nothing that cannot be corrected by
following the Way.

4

The Way is empty but not used up
The deep Way is like the root of all species

The Way blunts the sharp
The Way unties the trouble
The Way softens the glare
The Way harmonizes with the dust
The Way is dark, but it seems to exist

I do not know who the children of the Way are
But the Way appeared out before heaven and
earth.[6]

5

There is no kindness in heaven and earth
Consider all species like stray dogs
Heartless saints treat everyone like stray dogs
That exists between heaven and earth
Like a fire pipe
Empty but endless
The more intense the blow, the more intense the
dynamism

Many words contain little value
It is better to keep this in mind.[7]

6

The Way is the eternal breath
The Way is a woman
The woman is the mother of the beginning stage
The mother's gateway is the root of heaven and
earth
Like a veil very hard to see
Using the Way will never dry out.[8]

7

Heaven is undying
But why is it undying?
Because Heaven does not live for itself
Therefore, Heaven is undying

While the saint stands behind
People push to the front
The saint also stands outside
And gets along with everyone
When you act carefree,
The results will come.[9]

8

The perfect one is like water
Water provides life for all things
Without competing with anything
Water lives where people hate
Therefore, it can be compared with the Way

Accommodation is humble
Thinking is deep
Treatment is forgiven
Talking is genuine
Assertiveness is fair
Working is competent
Action is timely

When there's no contest, then there will be no mistakes.

9

Better to lack a little than be too full
When the sharpening knife is too sharp, it will
quickly become blunt
Houses are full of gold and pearls, are hard to keep
By pretending to be rich, one would harm himself

When you are done, you must retreat[10]
That is the Way of heaven.

10

By keeping body and soul together
Is it possible to keep them apart?
Pay attention to breathe
To be soft
Can one become an infant?
With spiritual cleansing
Can the stain be gone?
Love people and rule country
Can one without talent?
The heaven gate opens and closes
Can one become woman?
Through everything
Can't we do anything?

We are born and raised
Instructions without possessions
Made without merit
Instruction without ruling
Such is the root of the Way.

11

Thirty wood sticks make up a cart axle
Something empty becomes self-contained
Create the pot from the soil
The empty space of the pot is where people use
Cut the doors and windows to make the house
The empty space in the house is used for living

The existence of things is wealth
The non-existence of things is what to use.

12

Five colors make people's eyes blind
Five sounds make people's ears buzz
Five flavors make people's tongue lose taste
Chasing hunting horses makes people go crazy
Rare and precious possessions make one degrade
Sage prays for a full stomach
And yet there's nothing spectacular
Therefore, leave this and get that.

13

Be open to humiliation
What does "be open to humiliation" mean?
Accept bad luck like it's human destiny
Reception is not important
Do not worry about loss or gain
This is called "be open to humiliation"

What does "accept bad luck like it is human
destiny" mean?
Bad luck comes from one's body
If not, where does that bad fortune come from?

Be precious to one's body
As people believe one's body is everything
Love this world like one's body
Then one can fulfill everything.[11]

14

Look but not seeing because of formlessness
Listen but not hearing because of soundlessness
Get it but can't keep it because of being inanimate
Those three things cannot be traced
Because they are one

Above, do not illuminate
Underneath, do not overshadow
It is hard to describe something
When you are far away from it
Then back to nothing
The form of the formless
The shadow of the shadowless
That is called indescribable, non-visualizable

By standing in front, one can't see the head
By following, one can't see the tail
Keep the Way of the past in harmony with the present
Knowing primitiveness is the precept of the Way.

15

In ancient times, one skillfully practiced the Way
Delicately, mysteriously, profoundly, and
enthusiastically

They are deeply unpredictable
Because people can't guess
So people are forced to describe his looks
Cautious like one crossing the river in winter
Calm like one in times of danger
As polite as when welcoming guest
Soft as when ice melts into water
Rustic like untouched wood
Deep hollow like a cave
Nebulous like muddy water

Who can wait for the nebulous water to settle?
Who can remain still until the moment of action?

The Way users don't want to be filled
They don't want to be full
So one can change without being sacked.

16

Make it all empty
Keep your mind calm

All species born also pass away
Then they go back to the original source[12]
Returning to the origin is stillness
It is according to the law of nature
The natural law is immutable

Knowing the circulation of heaven and earth is
lucid
No knowing the circulation of heaven and earth is
dark

Knowing the circulation is lucid
By being lucid, then the soul is exuberant
By being exuberant, then the soul behaves fairly
Fairness is everywhere

Everywhere is suitable with nature
What is suitable with nature is suitable with the
Way

Being one with the Way is the true Way
Even when the body dies, the Way remains.

17

If the king is superior, the people only know the
people
When he is lower, the people love and praise
And lower than that, the people are afraid
Then at the lowest, the people are contempt

The sage says little
How does one value words by being quiet?

Work is accomplished
Things are done
People said: "They do it themselves."

18

When great Way is forgotten, benevolence appears
When wisdom and talent are born, lies appear
When the family is in conflict, a good man appears
When the country is in turmoil, loyal ministers
appear.[13]

19

By eliminating intellectual and discarding
knowledge,
People benefit a hundredfold
By eliminating humanity and discarding justice,
People are blessed
By eliminating artistry and discarding profit
Thieves and robbers are dissipated

These three things are external manifestations
They are not sufficient enough by themselves
And so should be more important
The outside keeps rustic
Keep yourself pure in mind
Be less esoteric
Then reduce longing.

20

Eliminate learning and worry less
What is the difference between good and evil?
Why are we scared of what others are afraid of?
So immense, it is impossible to know

Everyone is as cheerful as when enjoying a buffalo
feast
Like spring on the hill
I am silent alone
Like an infant who cannot yet laugh
Hanging down, walking like a homeless person

People have become redundant
I am destitute alone
My mind is like a fool
How dumb!
People are all bright and sharp
My own is dark and dull

People like the ocean's waves
Personally, I do not know which way the wind is
blowing

People are busy
My own boorish
I am different from people
I'm unlike other people
I trust in mother's milk to feed all species.

21

Great Virtue of practice is with the Way
The Way cannot be touched or captured
It cannot be touched or captured
But there's an image inside
It cannot be touched or captured
But there is a category inside[14]

The Way is dim
But inside has substance
This substance is very real
Which contains belief

From the primitive to the present
The Way is eternal
The Way is creation

How do we know that Way is the root of all
creatures?
That is why!

22

Concession is sure to win
Curvy is sure to straighten
Low is sure to full
Worn-out is sure to become new
Less is sure to more
More is sure to chaos

Sage embraces one to be an example for the world
By not showing off, one should shine like the sun
and moon
By not explaining away, one should stand out
Regardless, merit should be merited
By not being boastful, one should not be
embarrassed
Way is not a competition, so no one competes

Because the ancients said that concede is sure to
win
Then surely it is not an empty statement?
To be completely honest, everything will follow.

23

Nature is quiet

Strong wind does not blow the whole morning
Heavy rain does not fall all day
Why? Heaven and earth!
If heaven and earth can't do it
How can humans do it?

One with the Way
Then becomes one with the Way
One with Virtue
Then becomes one with Virtue
One who loses the Way and the Virtue
Then becomes one with loss

When one is one with the Way
The Way welcomes one
When one is together with the Virtue
The Virtue is always there
When one is together with loss
The loss also follows one

One who is disbelieved
Should not be believed.

24

Tiptoes cannot stand firm
Long steps do not go far
Ostentatious is not illuminant

Self-importance is not respected
Pompous does not achieve anything
Haughty cannot exist

The follower of the Way must stay away from the
above habits
Like leftover food
As unnecessary things.

25

There is a mystery taking shape
Born before heaven and earth
Quiet and empty
Stand alone without changing
Mobile forever without getting tired
Probably the mother of all species
I don't know what to call it
So temporarily, it is called the Way
Because of the lack of nouns
So it can also be called big

Because the Way is big
So you can be moving with it
Moving far away
Going far away, so come back

Therefore, "The Way is big
Heaven is big
Earth is big
Humans are also big"

Those are the four big things in the universe where
the human is one

Humans follow the earth
The earth follows heaven
Heaven follows the Way
The Way follows nature.

26

Heavy is the root of light
Static is the owner of the disturbance

The sage walks all day
Eyes do not leave the luggage
Though there is beauty to contemplate
But still self-controlled and calm

Why does the king hold ten of thousand soldiers
and consider the court very light?
Because light is to lose oneself
And acting heavy is to lose control.[15]

27

Skilled walker leaves no footprints
Skilled talker does not miss words
A skilled mathematician does not need a
comparison

Skillfully closed needs not locking
But no one can open it
Skillfully knotted needs not tied
But no one can remove it

Sage takes care of everyone
Not missing one
Sage takes care of everything
Nothing missing anything
That is called bright-hearted!

Who is a good person?
The teacher of the bad person
Who is the bad person?
Someone meant for the good person to teach

If the teacher is not respected
And the student does not love
Then there is confusion in talent
That is the pivotal point of the mystery.

28

Know the male and keep the female,
Making streams for people.
Making streams for people,
Virtue does not leave
Return to the childhood

Know the light and keep the dark,
Be an example for the world.
Be an example for the world,
Virtue does not leave
Return to infinite

Know the honor and keep the humiliation,
Make a cave for the world.
Make a cave for the world,
Virtue is full
Return to the rustic

Rustic is not divided
Sage uses it to provoke hundreds of officials

So the great spell is not undercut.

29

You want to bring people to reform?
I don't believe that is possible
People are holy
You cannot reform them
Change is awry
Keeping is lost

Sometimes things are in front, sometimes in the rear
Sometimes the wind is hot, sometimes cold
Sometimes strong, sometimes weak
People sometimes are above, and also sometimes below

The sage avoids excess, luxury, and complacency.

30

Those who use the Way to help the king
Do not rely on soldiers but submit to the world
Where the soldiers stomped, the thorns grew there
After winning a big battle, there must be a crop
failure

Skillful rescue only!
Do not rely on soldiers to be strong

Achieve results, not complacency
Not self-boasting, not elation
Because that is natural
When there is no violence

If you are losing power, then use violence
That is not the path of the Way
Acting opposite with the Way will soon be
destroyed.

31

Good weapons are ominous tools[16]
All species hate them
The gentleman respects the left side

The warmonger respects the right side
A weapon is an ominous tool
Gentlemen don't use it
It is only used for reluctance
Peace is a precious thing
Victory is not something to rejoice about
The one who rejoices in victory is a ferocious man
who likes to kill
By enjoying killing, one cannot satisfy people

Good works value to the left
Evil works value to the right
Vice general stands to the left
The general stands to the right
That is to take the funeral to judge

One should be grieving and sad because many
people die
That is why when victorious
One performs the funeral.

32

The Way is forever indefinable
It is small and formless
Not to hold on
If the king keeps it
All species obey
Heaven and earth bind
Drizzle rain falls
People do not need anyone to prevail but submit
themselves

Once the Way is divided, the name creates
When the name has enough
One would know how to stop
Know how to stop to avoid danger
The Way in the world like river water back to the
sea.

33

Knowing people is clever
Knowing oneself is lucid
Winning people is a strength
Winning oneself is potent

Knowing enough is wealth
Working hard is an ambition
Keeping yourself will last long
Death without loss is called longevity.

34

Great Way spreads everywhere
It moves to the left and moves to the right
It is depended on by everything
It creates without holding back
Work is accomplished, yet taking credit

The Way fosters all species without mastering
Without desire, it is called small
All species come back without mastering
And so are called great

In the end, the Way doesn't receive as great itself
That is why it accomplished a great thing.

35

By keeping the great Way, the people will follow
Because the Way is a comfortable and peaceful
place

Passersby stop for music and food
But talking about Tao is dull and tasteless
Look but seeing
Listen but hearing
But using it does not end.

36

Wanted contract, first stretch
Wanted weak, first strong
Wanted dump, first mania
Wanted receive, first give
It is: "The hidden object in the daytime"

Soft wins hard[17]
Big fish cannot leave the abyss
National vested interests cannot be displayed.

37

The Way does not act
But nothing is not done
If the king notices this
Then everything will change itself
If one wants to do
Be simple and rustic

Be invisible without desire
When there is no desire, then you will be
undisturbed
This is the path to self-healing.[18]

PART II

The Virtue

38

The highly virtuous people do not pray for virtue;
they already have virtue
The lowly virtuous people want virtue, so they
don't have virtue

The highly virtuous people do nothing
Yet nothing is undone
The lowly virtuous people always do
Yet many more things need to be done

The humane person works without letting the job
go unfinished
The righteous person works, but the undone jobs
are many
The polite person works, but no one responds

When the Way dies, the Virtue is born
When the Vitue dies, humanity is born
When humanity dies, the righteous is born
When the righteous die, the polite is born

Politeness is a shell of disloyalty
The clue of chaos
Using the mind to foresee flashes the Way
The clue of foolishness

Highly virtuous people live faithfully
They do not respect politeness
On the fruit, neither in the flower
One chooses this but leaves that.[1]

39

The old things are from One
Heaven is One; therefore, it is clear
The land is One; therefore, it is firm
The soul is One; Therefore, it is holy
The cave is One; therefore, it is full
Everything is One; therefore, they are alive
King is One; therefore, the world is righteous
This is called the Virtue of One[2]

Clear heaven prevents breaking
Firm land prevents cracking
Holy soul prevents dissipating
Full cave prevents drying up
Alive species prevents destruction
Righteous king prevents collapse

Wealth takes petty as the base
High takes low as a foundation
King sees himself as an orphan, widow, and also
useless
So is it petty as the base?
Isn't that so?
Therefore, being praised loses honor

Be non-vociferant as jade
It is better to be disdainful like pebbles.

40

Coming back is the acting of the Way
Birth is the effect of the Way
The Way produces all things
Being is born out of being.

41

Bright people who listen to the Way try hard to
execute
Ordinary people who listen to the Way are in doubt
Dark people who listen to the Way laugh
There is no Way without laughter

So the old saying goes
The bright Way seems to be dim
Forward seems to be backward
Seeing easy seems difficult

The highest Virtue seems empty
Clear seems to be cloudy
Broad Virtue seems helpless
Strong Virtue seems weak
Real Virtue seems virtual
The real square has no corners
Doing great things takes long
A high pitch is hard to hear
A large shape seems without form

The Way is hidden without a name
Only the Way has skillful birth and creation of all
things.

42

The Way gives birth to one
One gives birth to two
Two gives birth to three
Three gives birth to the universe[3]
Everything that carries negative holds positive
Combined, they are in harmony

The human hates orphan, widow, and useless ones
But the king sees himself as that
Therefore, his thoughts increase but also decrease
And then his thoughts decrease but also increase

The words that others and I promote are
"Violent man has brutal death!"
That is the main point I recommend.

43

The softest thing in the universe
Wins the hardest in the universe
Emptiness can get into space because there is a gap
So one knows the value of nothingness

Teaching without words is the benefit of inaction
Few people in this world can understand.

44

Fame or fate: Which is more important?
Fate or asset: Which is more valuable?
Gain or loss: Which one hurts more?

Ambition is a loss
Containing many, but loses much
Knowing enough is not disappointed
Knowing when to stop keeps one from danger
So one is forever sustainable.

45

Perfectly good seems lacking
Its use is unending
Fully full seems empty
Its use is inexhausting

Straight seems crooked
Wise seems stupid
Good reasoning seems awkward

Action restrains cold
Inaction restrains hot
Inaction is the natural state of the universe.

46

When people have the Way
Horses are used for farm work
When people do not have the Way
Warhorses are fighting outside the city

Catastrophy is nothing more than ignorance
Harm is nothing more than endless greed
Because who knows enough is always enough!

47

Do not go out but know the world
Do not look out the window but see the Way
The more one goes, the less one knows

So a sage does not go out but knows
Do not only look but see
Do not only do but accomplish.

48

Learn knowledge, then its increase
Learn the Way, then its decrease

Less, then more less
To reach the point of not doing
Because one does not do, so nothing is undone

People who follow the natural law
Can not be frustrated
If they are annoyed
The work will not be completed.

49

A sage does not have a heart of his own
He gets the heart of the world as his heart

One is good to good people
One is also good to those who are not good
Because the essence of Virtue is being good
One believes those who believe
One also believes those who do not believe
Because the essence of Virtue is believing

Sage in the world is carefree
He's in harmony with everyone
So people look and listen
But sage sees them as children.

50

Being born is called living
Coming back is called dead

Three-tenths live long
Three-tenths die prematurely
Three-tenths may live long but die early
Why?
Because they consider life is too heavy

People who know how to nourish life are not afraid
of rhinos or tigers
They fight without armor
Because rhino has no place to pierce horns
Tiger has no room to use its claws
The weapon has no room to penetrate
Why?
Because they don't fall into hazardous locations.[4]

51

The Way births
The Virtue nourishes
Thing shapes
Circumstances complete

Everything respects the Way and makes Virtue
precious
No one says to respect the Way or to make Virtue
precious
But that is the nature of all species

Therefore the Way births
Virtue keeps, nurtures, matures, ripes, protects and
buries

Born without receiving
Accomplish without holding
Raise without mastering
That is the miracle of Virtue.[5]

52

Everything has origin
At the beginning of everything is the mother of all
By keeping the mother, one knows the child
By knowing the child, one keeps the mother
Therefore, one should not be in danger for a
lifetime

Close-lipped, breath held
Life is full
Open-lipped, always busy[6]
Life is futile

Seeing hidden is bright
Hold strength is strong
Use Virtue to return to the Way
Do not let the body be in trouble
Thus, the Way is eternal.

53

If we have a little knowledge
One will walk on the main road and only fear losing
the path
Keeping the main road is easy
But people love the shortcut

When the court displayed its splendor
The farm fields are full of weed
The food warehouse is empty
Courtiers are displayed in luxurious dresses
Wearing a sharp sword
And eating excessively
Excess wealth
They are bandits
That is certainly not the road of the Way.

54

A skilled plant is difficult to eradicate
A skilled grasp is difficult to slip
Virtue will be honored from generation to
generation

By fixing Virtue in oneself, Virtue will be real
By fixing Virtue in the house, Virtue will have
redundancy
By fixing Virtue in the village, Virtue will grow
By fixing Virtue in the country, Virtue will be in
abundance
By fixing Virtue in the world, Virtue will be
everywhere

So, by oneself that considers others
By one's house that considers other houses
By one's village that considers other villages
By one's nation that considers other nations
By one's people that consider other people
How do we know what people are? Thanks for that!

55

People with deep Virtue like babies
Bees and snakes cannot spit poisonous nibs
Wild beasts cannot grab
Birds can't peck
Soft bones and weak tendons
But hold firm
Don't know how to have sexual intercourse
between men and women
But perfect vitality is living in abundance
Screaming all day but not hoarse
That is called harmony

Knowing the harmony is invariant
Knowing invariants is bright

Greed is catastrophe
Being greedy is not harmony
Disharmony is the opposite of the Way
The opposite of the Way is soon destroyed.[7]

56

Those who know don't say
Those who say don't know

Fill the hole
Close the door
Break the sharp
Unravel the tangle
Shield the bright
Mix with the dust
That is called being sociable

Who understands this state?
Then there is no longer a distinction between
friends or foes
Beneficial or harmful, noble or despicable
This is the most precious person in the world.[8]

57

Use the Way of truth to rule the country
Use surprise to attack in battle
Do not fight but subdue the people

How do we know that?
Because of this:
The more the laws forbid, the more the poor people
become
The sharper the weapon,
The more turmoil the country becomes
The more the talented people cause mischief
The more laws, the more robbers

So sage:
One does nothing, but people transform themselves
One is at ease, but the world is pure
One gives the laws, but people become rich
One does not pray for lust, but people return to
rustic.[9]

58

Politics blurred, the people are mere
Politics clearly, the people are cunning

Disaster is the fulcrum of blessing
Blessing hides under the shadow of disaster
Who can understand how disaster and blessing
are?
They are not in a certain direction
Honesty becomes lying
Goodness becomes suspicious
Humans have been in a sodden for a long time!

So sage:
Be sharp without hurting
Just without harming
Straight without offending
Bright without blinding.

59

In caring for others and worshiping god
There is nothing like restraint
Restraint begins with giving up one's will
This belongs to Virtue gained from experience
If you store a lot of Virtue, nothing can be undone
If there is nothing one can't undo, then there's no
restraint
If there is no restraint, then one can cure the
country
Knowing the root of country treatment is long-
lasting
That is called deeply-rooted, durable descent
That is the Way to live long and see throughout.

60

Treating a big country is like cooking a baby fish

If a sage uses the Way
Then the devil will not be efficacious
And deity can't harm people either
Not only can deity not harm people
Nor do sages harm people
The two sides do not harm each other
So Virtue keeps coming back.[10]

61

The big country seems to be located in low land
That is the gathering place of all species
The mother of all things

Females prevail over males due to their stillness
Take stillness as a low place

Therefore, if a big country is humble with a small
country
Then it will conquer the small country
If a small country is humble with a big country
Then it will be protected by the big country
So staying below to get it
Or staying below to be protected

A big country wants to accommodate many people
The small country needs many people to
accommodate
Each side gets what they want
So the big country should learn to be humble.

62

The Way is the root of all species
A treasure of good people
A place of refuge for bad people

Sweet words can buy fame
Doing good deeds can add respect
But if it's a bad person, why quit?

So on the day the king is crowned
To appointing three ministers
Two hands offered jade in front of the four-horse
carriage
Better by kneeling in the mud to pray for the Way

Why do people in ancient times like the Way?
Is it not what one is looking for?
And if guilty, will one be forgiven?
So the Way is the most precious to people.

63

Act without moving
Do without getting your hands embedded
Taste the tasteless
Increase the small
Make extra the few

Plan the hard work while still easy
Plan the big work while small or not yet present
Hard work in the world
It surely starts from easy
Big work in the world
Surely starts from small

Sages are not doing the big
So they accomplish the big

Few believe in empty promises
They despise things and face difficulty
Sage considers everything difficult
Therefore, no trouble.[11]

64

Stillness is easy to grasp
Formlessness is easy to plan
The crispiness is easy to break
Small pieces are easy to disperse
Prevent at, yet present
Treat at, yet chaos starts

Big tree as one hug
They are born from a small seed
A nine-story high floor
It is erected from a crate of soil
Walking thousands of miles away
But starting with the first step

One who acts, fails
One who holds loses
Therefore:
Sage doesn't act
Thereupon he doesn't fail
Doesn't keep
Thereupon he doesn't lose

Things often fail when they are about to be
accomplished
Because not as cautious as at first
If the following caution is used as before, the job
will not fail

So the sage avoids ambition
Or precious desire
He just wants to teach the uneducated
Help bring people back to the Way
Help things grow naturally
Therefore, one should not interfere with anything.

65

The sage of the past did not use the Way to
enlighten the people
Only use the Way to make people honestly emanate

People of plots are difficult to rule
If one uses wit to govern the people, one will harm
the country
If one does not use wit to govern the people, one
will bless the people

Understanding these two things is understanding
the law of heaven
Through these two spells, it is called legend Virtue
Legend Virtue is deep
Then everything is back to the original
They are in compliance with nature.[12]

66

Rivers and seas are the kings of hundreds of
streams
Because you should be smart by staying in the
lower place
If one wants to be in the higher places in the world
One has to say humble words
If one wants to stand before the world
One has to step back

Therefore, sage:
Above, but people do not feel heavy
In front, but people do not feel obscured
So people worship without knowing boredom

Because there was no contest
So no one contested.[13]

67

People say my Way is very big
There is nothing like the Way
If so, the Way is already small

There are three treasures that I always carefully
hold by my side:
One is benevolence[14]
Second is frugality[15]
Third is not daring to stand in front of people

Benevolence should produce courage
Frugality should produce affluence
Do not dare to stand in front of people, so by praise;
you become the master of the people

Give up benevolence to be brave
No frugality to be affluent
Do not stand behind but master the world
One certainly must die!

By taking benevolence to fight, you will surely win
By taking benevolence to defend, you will surely
secure

Heaven wants to save someone
Then gives benevolence to help him.

68

A good fighter does not use aggression in martial
arts
A good fighter does not get angry
A smart winner is not fighting directly with the
enemy
A smart leader puts himself below

Someone with virtue does not contest
He is called someone with virtue who knows how
to use the strength of others
So that is completely suitable with the Way.

69

Conducting a war has a saying:
One does not dare to be a master
But just want to be a guest
One does not dare to advance one inch
But just wants to take a foot back
That is advancing without contest
Set a battle without having to raise your arm
Capture the enemy without having to use a weapon
Winning the enemy is like going into an empty
space[16]

Nothing is more dangerous than the
contemptuousness of the enemy
Contemptuousness of the enemy will lose many
treasures like fallen leaves on a branch
So when fighting
The benevolence side will win.[17]

70

My words are easy to understand, easy to practice
But people do not understand
Therefore people do not practice

My words have the root
My job is well-structured
Because people do not understand me
So they don't know me

People who understand me are very little
People who follow me are rare
So the sage wears the rough cloth
But the heart embraces precious jewels.

71

Knowing the unknown is superior
Not knowing but pretending to know is wrong

Of course, one must not know the wrong thing
Because knowing the wrong thing is a disease
Therefore, one shouldn't get sick.

72

When people are not afraid of power
Then the king must be scared of his power

Do not bother with people's lives
Do not bother with the people's work
If the people are not bothered, they do not bother
the king

The sage knows himself; therefore, he is not
showing off
The sage keeps Virtue to himself; therefore, he is
not proud
So one leaves the latter and keeps the former.

73

A brave one who greedily fights must die
A brave one who is calm must live
Those two things are important:
One births, and one dies
Be very careful
Even a sage also thinks it is difficult

Heavenly Way is not contested but won
Do not say but respond well
Do not call, but things come
Quiet but clever plan

The net is sparse
However scatter, it is difficult to pass.[18]

74

People are not afraid of death
Why use death to scare?
If it makes people always afraid
And if every criminal is caught and killed
So who is left?

Killing is carried out by the executioner
Replace that person
Like replacing a woodcutter
Which rarely cuts hands.

75

Heavy taxes make people hungry
And the people are hard to rule because the law is
too strict

People despise death
Because the rulers are harsh

Only people who live are not too extreme
Their lives are precious.

76

Newborn humans are pliable
When they are dead, they are stiff
Newly born trees are soft
When they are dead, they are hard and dry.

So stiff and hard represent death
Pliable and softness represent life
Strong and violent is the dead
Hard trees are cut

So hard and strong should be put under
Pliable and softness should be put above.

77

The Way of heaven is like stretching a bow high,
Then lowering the bow low
Then raising the bow again
Abate the surplus
Fill the lack

The Way of the people are not so
Abate the lack
Fill the surplus

Who knows how to take the surplus and give it to
the world?
Only a Way person can do that!

So sages do without relying on success
They do without contesting
They do not show self-ingenuity.

78

Under the dome of the sky, nothing is softer than
water
But the hard-hitting attack is nothing more
So nothing can replace it[19]

Weak wins strong
Soft wins hard
Everyone knows
But no one can follow

So sage:
By withstanding the stains of the home country
Then he can master the nation
By withstanding the disasters of the people
Then he can be the king of the people[20]

Straight words sound like a contradiction.

79

Solve big enmity
Yet small enmity exists
So why is it so?

So sage:
Keep the contract on the left
Without harassment

Those with Virtue keep the terms of the treaty
A non-virtuous person takes it all

Heaven Way is not biased
But always stands by the people with the Virtue.[21]

80

A small country has a small population
Although there are many means
But still no need for those

People value death
So they don't move far away from their families

There are boats and carts
But no need to use them
There are armors and weapons
But they are not on display

Make people use the knot style again
Food is simple but delicious
Cloth is rudimentary but beautiful
The house is primitive but peaceful
Tradition is pure but fun

So the neighboring countries see each other
Hear each other's chickens crowing and dogs
barking
But when they are dying in old age
They are still not going back and forth with each
other.[22]

81

The truthful words are not gaudy
The gaudy words are not the truth
Good people do not argue
The people that argue are not good
People who know are not broad-minded
The broad-minded people do not know

The sages do not hoard
The more one helps others; the more one has a surplus
The more one gives others, the more one has

The Way of Heaven expands without hindering
The Way of sage does without contesting.[23]

Notes

Part I: The Way (Chapter 1 to Chapter 37)

1. Way is the path that people follow, sending all things to act but its origin is the mystery. Way is the universal law of the universe, governing all species.

2. Whenever a noun is used to designate something, the specified object has been limited. Since Way is absolute, there is nothing to compare.

3. The body of Way is "non-being", extremely magical. The use of Way is "being", extremely great.

4. These verses use the law of criticism in life, the purpose is only to advise us to be calm before everything. Only then will the mind be quiet.

5. Lao Tzu said that lust is the focal point of the chaos. He thinks that people just need to eat enough, be healthy, pure, and have no desire, by then the society will naturally be autonomous.

6. The application of the Way is both an entity and a void, taking it all, using it, and being extremely flexible. Because Way is naturally infinite, being mystery everywhere. Its body is hard to find and the act is hard to realize.

7. The Way creates all species naturally. The world should behave according to natural reason, then everything is in the right place. The society will be peaceful and happy.

8. Because the body of the Way is nothingness, so it covers, contains, biochemistry and nurture all species without ever running out.

9. A saint reaches to a sublime position because he takes other men's job for his work; put other people things first.

10. "When done, retreat" is synonymous with the folk saying: "Success, the body withdraws."

11. Hold a position without leaving it, behave in a righteous way without changing hearts, see doubts without indiscriminate acceptance, see benefits without taking it indiscriminately, the person with the above conditions is a master.

12. Everything moves in opposite directions: leaving and returning. To return is to go to the source, to be pure and also to be with the Way.

13. When all things live by nature, without humans intervening, there is no forced force, there is no reason to practice humanity, manner, intellectual, filial piety, loyaly. These things violate the nature of mankind and arise only in opposition to a dishonest society.

14. There is nothing more enlightened by considering the substance of the matter inside.

15. To do our best to listen to the will of the people, lose the autonomy to obey the will of the people.

16. Those who have the Way never earnestly raise soldiers, use force. If you have to use it, even if you win or lose, many people will die in the battlefield. That is a misfortune for the world.

17. The Way and worldly knowledge are very different, so Lao Tzu uses the first 4 contrasting sentences with the title "Soft wins hard".

18. Even to the Way, I do not want. Not wanting it because I have immersed myself in the Way. Way and I are one. That is the real Way. If I still desire Way that means Way is different from me and I am outside of Way. That means Way is like an obstacle to me. So neither does Way ever bother.

Part II: The Virtue (Chapter 38 to Chapter 81)

1. This chapter captures Lao Tzu's principles. He took "nameless" as Way and "named" as Virtue, belongs to the being, then the order from virtue down to human, manner, ceremony, wisdom. The lower the worst, the far away. Heaven and earth gave birth to all things, and the earth was very large but heaven and earth have never claimed to be virtuous. All things also do not know the virtue of heaven and earth. That is why there is no need of virtue, no need of accepting virtue, and no need of knowing virtue. So there is perfect, transcendent virtue. Actually, according to Lao Tzu, heaven and earth do nothing, but nothing they won't created. All living creatures that are in heaven and earth never need to intervene or self-acknowledge. It is because of not doing, so there is nothing to do, nor nothing, because nature does it.

2. Virtue is what people have in themselves, embrace everything that they all have their own will (Virtue is the divine power of the saints, so that whatever they do, they can easily succeed).

3. Way can't be seen. One is body, two is yin and yang, and three is yin and yang in harmony. When yin and yang are in harmony, they create all things.

4. As human, everyone is greedy to live and fear death. But the greed of life makes people blind, foolish, shorten their life and dig their own bury. Because outside, we let the matter destroy, inside we let the lust to burn, for our fellow human beings, we are jealous and contested. Isn't that just yourself rushing into swords, tigers, rhinos?

5. Way is the body of virtue. Virtue is the use of Way. So body is Way and the use of Way is Virtue. Therefore, the use of Way is very deep and mysterious.

6. The more ones say the more wrongs one gets. The more one does the more wrongs one gets.

7. Tô Triệt discussed that Lao Tzu, when it comes to morality, often uses children as an example, which is to say that. Oh! Children have foreign objects coming but do not know how to react, so they cannot talk about use. It is inherently silent, quite, and without lust. Its body is very innocent. People have a mind and then they have an image. There must be a collision with other objects that oppose us. The hurt doesn't tell the end. Only a child is heartless, does not confront external things. Ask which way does it hurt? It does not hold, but self-holds firmly. It

does not desire but acts on its own, reacts. It's because it's redundant, not because of its mind. If the mind has moved, the qi will be damaged, but screaming must lead to loss of hoarseness. Now it screams all day but is still at ease, just because its mind is not moving and its qi is calm. If you draw, don't let the outside harm the inside. Knowing peace is called normal, so it can keep the root to deal with everything around. On the contrary, it greatly increases life, making it impossible for qi to react according to the natural path. People are getting stronger and stronger, trying their best, then old age will follow. That is to lose the nature of the child.

8. Tô Triệt said: things can be close to them, they can be cold, and they can be noble and they can be mean. The human being is in harmony with the Tao, encompassing all things evenly, so that nothing is close or far away. He considers both favorable and unfavorable circumstances, happiness as well as suffering, so there are no problems. I don't know what is honor and what is shame, so there are no people who appreciate convenient people. All relativity is left out of the circle of feeling. Therefore, being in the world is very high and luxurious.

9. Trương Mặc Sinh said: Those who fix the country's affairs, the eyes must see far, see wide, plan eternal things, so they do not use the artificial but use the main. Soldiers are unpredictable and dangerous things, the holy man only temporarily copes with temporary events. That's why it was said, "make country justice and use tricks to control the military affairs." However, to bring

justice to the country, one must be in accordance with the Tao. But it is still a conditioned way of rule, can only keep one country, but taking the whole world is definitely not possible. Therefore, it is said to bring "nothing to get the world." Nothing means empty, no action, no arrangement of work. To hold is to take, here it means to hold to fix, arrange to change. That is to make people naturally act according to the Tao, by the way of unconditioned.

10. This chapter borrows the cooking of baby fish to compare it with the correction of a great nation. Cooking baby fish should not be contemptuous of stirring. Repairing large countries should not be too much work, too much changes. There is not much to change, that is, only putting one's heart into following the natural transformation, applying the "correction without doing anything." In this way, heaven and earth, ghosts and spirits, all things, and the world will all be in peace, without harming each other. Virtue will join together to make peace and return to One.

11. This chapter is about the natural way of keeping Way naturally. Only those who keep the Way for big, small, few and many can be considered equal. Only those who keep their Way behave of favor or revenge contrary to the common sense of the world. When it comes to plotting difficult things from easy, and doing big things from small, only those who keep the Way, know the roots, can understand the meaning of the easy and the small.

12. People follow the Way just like the water flows down low, flowing smoothly. The leader

instructs the people, although the people do not understand it, they can still follow it. When they understand and have enjoyed the true taste of the Way, they will dance and stomp their feet; naturally joyfully enlightened.

13. The king does not self humble, the world will not compete well with him. The king does not boast, the world will not compete with the king. The king must behave in such a way that everyone knows that there is a king above and in front of everyone, then people will happily honor the king to sit on and stand in front.

14. Good heart comes from the mind. That is the use of Way. For example, when a child's life is in danger. Mother dares to sacrifice her life to save the child. What other strength is there than the strength that radiates from the bottom of a mother's heart?

15. Hàn Phi Tử argues that a wise scholar who uses thrift will get rich. A sage who knows how to take care of the spirit will be full of spirit and not be damaged. The master knows that the soldiers' lives are precious, the population will increase day by day and the country will expand more and more, in short, wealth, fullness of spirit, large population, vast country, abundant and full life. All due to one word: saving!

16. Owner is against, guest is favorable; tired owners, cavalier guests; forward is arrogance, backward is humility; to move forward is to be impatient and agitated, to retreat is to be gentle and quiet. Take advantage of waiting for tired enemy; take rest, wait for pride; get quiet and wait for

impatiently. Such strength is the invincible power. That army went without a battle; twist shirt without using arms; wield weapons like no weapons; capture the enemy without fighting enemy. The above points show us what it is to win without fighting, like bringing troops into an empty place.

17. Because the saint knows pain and suffering, he appreciates everyone, making the whole people eager to rise up. So, definitely defeat the enemy. That is why it is said: so when fighting, the side with sincerity will win.

18. Nguy Nguyên explained that: strong in dare to do will often pay attention to the point of killing and not letting go. Strong in not daring to do, will often focus on the point of preserving people's lives. In the two lines, both use the strong, but the advantage and the disadvantage, are divided into two. It is impossible not to scrutinize. Why? Because people are strong in the daring to kill and because they are obedient to God's anger and hatred, so they are determined to practice without thinking that it is difficult at all. But God's will is deep, who knows for sure who is really being hated by God. Therefore, even saints obey God's orders to punish sins, but from the penalty of killing, they do not dare to disdain. God gives birth to all things like parents give birth to children, born without ever having the heart to destroy. Timely until an object rushes to find its way to death, even if it wants to save it, it can't be done, so the net is tilted upside down. It proves that the net of the heaven is thin, though it is sparse, but it does not let any hairs out. Why

does heaven need to borrow people from the world to keep their blessings?

19. Breaking hard is nothing better than hammer and fire. Although hard as iron, stone can't stand it. But hammer and fire alone are no better than water. On the contrary, it is also eroded, crushed and extinguished by water.

20. King Câu Tiến suffered disgrace for his country. King Lê Lợi during the reign of the Ming Dynasty, for the sake of his country, suffered disasters and tribulations when he lost the battle, his family was separated, Lê Lai had to die for him instead.

21. Trương Mặc Sinh argued that: having great resentment, only worrying about reconciliation to dissolve, of course, it is inevitable that there will be some residual resentment, so is that not a good solution? Therefore, saints often keep the piece on the left side of the contract without asking or demanding from others. Saying this means that the saint corrects the world, the owner is in "doing nothing but ruling", so he only holds the piece on the left side of the contract, prays that it is enough to be consistent with the faith, does not bear harsh demands and demands on humanity people. Then there will be peace between the top and bottom, right from the start, resentment has no reason to arise, let alone resentment and wait for resolution. Therefore, the virtuous king often held the left side of the contract, determined not to disturb the masses. The new ungodly king advocated setting up many laws, using many methods of destruction and killing at will to show his will to the nation. But the way of heaven does not

only love people, but only always helps virtuous people, unscrupulous people should examine themselves and be alert.

22. Hà Giám Tôn said that a small country with small population borders close to a large country with big population, although it is difficult to govern, if one can follow the use of the Way and strive to keep the nation from being disturbed because of skillful occupations, strange, profanity, then even though many sharp tools, ten times more powerful than human strength, still can not use for anything. The things that need to be used are only plows, harrows, and hoes, which make people satisfied with their lives, their possessions are usually full. Therefore, they naturally value death and do not want to leave their dwelling place; respecting death for the sake of living and not relocating because of a peaceful business; born in any land where it is enough to live in that land, although having boats and vehicles, they do not have to ride or sit on. There are no fighting comics, no theft inside, no resentment against neighbors outside. Armor and military equipments are purchased enough but not worn, use, and displayed. The goverment doesn't push taxes for many, the people doesn't file a lawsuit. Simple rustic customs, almost nothing to do. People can just tie the rope to record the job is enough. Eating their own chestnut, barley is delicious because of their own transplant. Wearing a raw cotton fabric, beautiful because of their own weaving. Not asking for the five scents and colors to cause confusion, so the people live in peace and quiet, enjoying the customs, although the neighboring countries can be seen and heard

by each other clearly of the sound of roosters crowing and dogs barking, but no one intends to move. In the country, there is no practice of soldiers wearing armor, hunting animals, or stationing posts. People do not interact with each other until old age and death. It is not forbidden by anyone, but because of the need for daily communication, the story of wandering in the battlefield or fleeing from the war is even more absent. Everyone who has tools that they don't use, has boats and ships that don't go, has armor that they don't wear, all because of their beliefs, naturally become like this, not because of the law. Rusticism has turned into a routine, people will find that they eat well, dress well, stay still, and be happy with their lifestyle. The sage corrects, the effect is clearly visible. When the old way of life has become familiar, the story of "hanging clothes, clasping hands, everyone is at peace" is no longer a myth or a fantasy.

23. Tiêu Hanh explained: people can enjoy Lao Tzu's books and see beauty; seeing that in the end, there is nothing wrong with the logic of all things, as if it were close to the rebuttal and the vast understanding. However, they do not know that there is something else - true faith but not beauty, good without refuting, knowing but not learning widely - lies within. What does it mean? That's because what is said in five thousand words is the Way that is not contained, stored, or empty. By not contained, stored or empty then the heart is not bound, imprisoned. One speaks without saying so! However, it's not that we don't work for people but we don't compete, so we never separate of what we "have"; not without

giving it to others, but never making to self that we already have much to be consumed. Then why hate rebuttal, hate studying widely? Just because you keep holding on to your opinions to compete with the rest of the world, you are in the category of "the more you talk, the more its consumed you" - not the way of heaven. If the scholar who understands the above in his heart to forget the five thousand words in this book, then Tao Te Ching already understood more than half.

Further Readings

1. Bukkyo Dendo kyokai, *The Teaching Of Budda*, Society For Promotion Of Buddhism, 1995.

2. Chang Chung Yuan, *Original Teachings Of Ch'an Buddhism*, Grove Press, Inc., 1969.

3. David Scott, Tony Doubleday, *The Elements Of Zen*, Barns & Noble, Inc., 1997.

4. Đào Duy Anh, *Việt Nam Văn Hóa Sử Cương*, T.P. Hồ Chí Minh, 1992.

5. Eckhart Tolle, *The Power of Now*, New World Library and Namaste Publishing, 1999.

6. Ellen M. Chen, *The Tao Te Ching*, Paragon House, 1989.

7. Giáp Văn Cường, *Lão Tử: Đạo Đức Huyền Bí*, Đồng Nai, 1995.

8. John Heider, *The Tao Of Leadership*, Batam Books, 1988.

9. Kim Định, *Việt Lý Tố Nguyên*, An Tiêm, 2001.

10. Lý Tế Xuyên, *Việt Điện U Linh Tập*, Translated by Lê Hữu Mục, Khai Trí, 1960.

11. Man-Ho Kwok, Martin Palmer, Jay Ramsay, *Tao Te Ching*, Barns & Noble Books, 1993.

12. Michael Reagan, *The Holy Bible*, Illuminated Family Edition, Skyhorse Publishing, 2000.

13. Nghiêm Toản, *Lão Tử Đạo Đức Kinh*, Khai Trí, 1971.

14. Nguyễn Duy Cần, *Lão Tử Tinh Hoa*, Đại Nam.

15. Nguyễn Hiến Lê, *Luận Ngữ*, Văn Học, 1994.

16. Nguyễn Hiến Lê, *Mặc Học*, Văn Hóa, 1995.

17. Nguyễn Hiến Lê, *Trang Tử Và Nam Hoa Kinh*, Văn Hóa – Thông Tin, 1994.

18. Nguyễn Hiến Lê, *Tuân Tử*, Văn Hóa, 1994.

19. Nguyễn Hồng Trang, *Trang Tử: Trí Tuệ Của Tự Nhiên*, Đồng Nai, 1995.

20. Nguyễn Hữu Liêm, *Tự Do Và Đạo Lý*, Biển Mới, 1993.

21. Phạm Văn Sơn, *Việt Sử Toàn Thư*, Khai Trí, 1972.

22. Nguyễn Văn Trương, Đinh Kim Quốc Bảo, *Từ Điển Anh-Anh-Việt*, Văn Hóa Thông Tin, 2008.

23. Phanxicôxavie Nguyễn Văn Thuận TGM, *Đường Hy Vọng*, Spes-Divine Compassion Publications, 1991.

24. Phùng Quý Sơn, *Mạnh Tử*, Đồng Nai, 1995.

25. Ralph Alan Dale, *Tao Te Ching*, Fall River Press, 2002.

26. Ray Grigg, *The Tao Of Relationships*, Batam Books, 1988.

27. Tư Mã Thiên, *Sử Ký*, Translated by Phan Ngọc, Văn Hóa Thông Tin, 1999.

28. Vũ Kim Biên, *Văn Hiến Làng Xã Vùng Đất Tổ Hùng Vương*, Trung Tâm UNESCO Thông Tin Tư Liệu Lịch Sử Và Văn Hóa Việt Nam và Cơ Sở Văn Hóa Thông Tin Thể Thao Phú Thọ, 1999.

29. William Scott Wilson, *Tao Te Ching*, Shambhala Publicattions, Inc., 2012.

Lao Tzu 老子